The s

The powerful healing of Autophagy uses your bodies natural intelligence to promote anti aging .Learn how to initiate it through extended water, Intermittent fasting & more

Naomi William & Rachel Pilon

Table of Contents

Chapter 1: Introduction

Autophagy is a process by which the body's cells recycle their components. Autophagy is one of those processes that run silently without us knowing it is going on. There are times when the level of autophagy increases to keep you safe, especially when you are under a lot of stress.

Autophagy is a term borrowed from Greek literature, meaning self-eating. It is a self-regulating process where body cells do away with toxic foreign or damaged components. These cell components are recycled by the cells to serve different purposes.

Autophagy is a homeostatic process. It regulates and maintains the level of protein in your body cells, preventing a buildup of toxic waste products. It also helps to remove pathogens and maintain proper function of the organelles. When you are starving or fasting, it is through autophagy that the body can sustain itself from the most basic level, the cellular level.

While a lot of studies have been conducted into autophagy over the years, in 2016 Yoshinori Ohsumi was awarded the Nobel Prize in Physiology or Medicine for the discoveries he had made in the mechanisms for autophagy. This was a sign that the advancements made in autophagy were ready to take center stage in modern medicine. Because autophagy has been proposed as a means to an end for so many diseases and ailments, there is promise for managing or finding a cure for things like cancer.

What happens in autophagy is that the autophagosome collects all the cell components and moves them to the lysosome where they are broken down into smaller parts that can be recycled into new components. Autophagy is carried out through ATG (autophagy-related genes). Autophagosome is initiated by the VPS34 complex and involves the ATG8 proteins and ATG9. Other components involved are the ATG12, ATG16L1, and ATG5.

There are genes in the body that detect any changes that take place at the cellular level. These genes turn autophagy on or off when they detect any changes within the cell structure. The mTOR genes monitor the nutrient level in the cells and prevent the VPS34 complex from forming by disrupting ULK1, especially when the body is receiving a lot of nutrients.

Cellular energy level is monitored by AMPK to determine the amount of ATP present, and it initiates autophagy when your energy level is low. The oxygen level in the body is monitored by HIF1A, whose target is the mitochondria, and initiates hypoxia by turning on autophagy.

Types of Autophagy

Since the beginning of the study of autophagy, researchers have come up with three main types of autophagy, namely microautophagy, macroautophagy, and chaperone-induced autophagy. By studying the types of autophagy, it is easier to get an in-depth perspective of the role that autophagy plays in the body, and how cellular functions are affected.

Microautophagy

Microautophagy is a process where the lysosome takes up the cytosolic components on its own. This takes place through the lysosome membrane. In simpler terms, microautophagy is the direct absorption of particulate or soluble cell components into the lysosomes. It is a degradative process where the cytoplasm cargo is engulfed directly at the boundary membranes through autophagic tubes responsible for vesicle scission and invagination into the lumen. Microautophagy can be initiated by rapamycin or through nitrogen starvation. The main functions of microautophagy include membrane homeostasis, maintaining the organelle size and ensuring cellular survival in a period of nitrogen starvation.

Macroautophagy

Macroautophagy is the process where cells surround a portion of cytoplasm by forming autophagosomes, double-membrane vesicles. Over time the autophagosomes bind to the lysosomes, degenerating their components in the process. While mammalian cells experience macroautophagy at the cellular level on a regular basis, it is often initiated by stressful situations like starvation.

There are several substrates of macroautophagy, including cytosolic proteins, damaged organelles, and microbes. After degradation, the products that are broken down are moved back to the cytosol, recycling the molecular components and providing energy to keep the cells functioning even when the body is under duress or an unfavorable condition.

Chaperone-Mediated Autophagy

Chaperone-mediated autophagy (CMA) is a catabolic pathway that supports the degrading of specific subsets of cytosolic proteins within lysosomes. In this process chaperone proteins like HSC-70 translocate the specific proteins through lysosome membranes; hence it is an intracellular catabolic pathway.

While lysosomes often randomly degrade cellular cytosol, it is also possible that they can target specific cytosol components for degradation, especially when a degradation tag is involved. Recent studies have shown that CMA is responsible for modulating DNA repair, lipid and glucose metabolism, and cellular responses to stress. Therefore, CMA, which was initially assumed to help in protein quality control, has been shown to have a physiological relevance. Things like cancer and neurodegeneration as a result of aging can be attributed to the failure in chaperone-mediated autophagy.

Autophagy is also responsible for killing some cells when the conditions are right. This process is referred to as programmed cell death (PCD) or autophagic cell death. The process of autophagic cell death is what experts refer to as apoptosis. There are different pathways and mediators responsible for apoptosis, making autophagy a nonapoptotic programmed cell death.

What autophagy does is to maintain a homeostatic balance between the production of cellular components and breaking down of cellular components and organelles that have been deemed surplus to requirements, or those that are damaged.

Ultimately, autophagy is simply a process where the body cleanses and detoxifies itself. While the body can initiate autophagy on its own, there are benefits to eating right and encouraging the body to initiate autophagy more frequently. Some of these benefits include the following:

- **Improved skin tone**

Everyone hopes to have great skin tone and quality for years to come. You can only achieve this by activating autophagy earlier in life. There are so many toxins that we come across as we go through the daily challenges or struggles in life.

The skin is the largest organ in the body. It has millions of pores, which are entry and exit points for toxins into the body. By activating autophagy, you encourage the body to eliminate toxins from the body, in the process helping you improve and maintain the ideal skin tone.

- **Slows down the aging process**

As you grow older, the body becomes less effective in performing certain tasks. Aging is a natural process. Think about aging like regular house cleaning. If you clean your house often, you barely have to worry about dirt building up. However, most people like to wait until the house is too dirty and they cannot avoid it; then they perform a thorough cleaning.

Autophagy is like house cleaning. If you perform it regularly, you will barely have to worry about cleaning the house. Your system will be functioning perfectly most of the time. It becomes easier for you to fend off diseases and illnesses because the body is always alert. In the long run, you slow down the process of aging.

- **Reduce inflammation**

Most health conditions and chronic diseases can be traced back to inflammation. Considering some of the poor dietary decisions and lifestyle choices that we make from time to time today, it is no secret that inflammation is one of the things you have to worry about.

Inflammation can also come about as a result of poor sleep patterns, or increased exposure to environmental toxins in your environment. The first step toward protecting you from diseases and improving your wellness and health is to reduce inflammation. This is one of the primary roles of autophagy.

You can make a few changes in your life to initiate autophagy. Activating autophagy is a simple process, and can be done in the following ways:

- **Intermittent fasting**

Since the body no longer receives the food it needs to digest and generate energy, it has to reach within its depths to source the energy. The body looks within the cells to find components that can be recycled to produce the energy it needs.

- **Eating more healthy fats**

Keeping a high fat, low carb diet forces the body to find other sources of fuel since it is not getting sufficient carbs to burn glucose. The body, therefore, resorts to burning fat. This is the same thing that happens when you are fasting or starving. It is what induces detoxification, cleansing, and autophagy. Therefore, having more healthy fats in the body than carbs initiates autophagy.

- **Activating the lymphatic system**

The body's lymphatic system is its natural detoxifier. It can be manually activated through exercise, or mundane things like taking a cold or hot shower, deep breathing, being in a sauna or anything that initiates excess sweating.

- **Being active**

Being active works in the same way as activating the lymphatic system. Activity increases the flow of blood, sends more oxygen to the body cells, and improves your blood circulation, making the body more efficient.

- **Sleeping**

So much goes on in the body without your knowledge. When you are asleep, your body detoxifies, repairs and recovers from the damage that its cellular components have been exposed to through the day. This is also the time when autophagy takes place. If you are not sleeping, the body does not get enough time to restore itself, so autophagy does not take place as often as it should.

Given the right environment, resources and nutrients, your body can perform all the tasks needed to keep you healthy. However, with a little help here and there, you can push your body further, encouraging optimal functions and living a better, healthier life.

Chapter 2: History of Autophagy

Autophagy is a science that is currently fronted by many nutritionists and physicians for different reasons. Most people who follow celebrity lifestyles come across autophagy a lot. A lot of celebrities embark on autophagy to lose weight to suit a specific role in a very short time. However, autophagy is not a new concept. This is a study that has matured over the years.

The year 2018 marks the 55th anniversary of Christian de Duve introducing the term *autophagy*[1], in reference to the process of degradation of cytoplasmic components within the vacuole or lysosome. After his discovery of lysosomes, studies into electron microscopy would later reveal that autophagy could help deliver intracellular constituents to the lysosomes.

At a molecular level, it was a long time before any studies were able to produce relevant advances in an attempt to understand the fundamental pathway of degradation. In the early 1990s, a yeast study revealed the concept of autophagy. The microscopic observation was made in yeast subject to starvation.

---

[1] From Christian de Duve to Yoshinori Ohsumi: More to Autophagy than just dining at home https://www.ncbi.nlm.nih.gov/pubmed/28411887

The problem of autophagy was not fully understood, and therein existed many misconceptions. Many defective mutants were discovered in light of a genetic effort to understand some of the misconceptions and problems of autophagy. Here we look at some of the historical advances that have been made in the field of autophagy over the years.

Autophagy, also referred to as *self-eating*[2], is a unique cellular pathway that influences the degradation of organelles and proteins. Autophagy also plays an important role in homeostasis, development, and survival. Research into autophagy started in the 1950s, but most activity has been experienced in this field in the past 20 years. Autophagy is useful to human health, given that it also influences human physiology, lifespan and the development of slowing down of diseases including cancer.

Autophagy is coined from a Greek word, *phagy*, which means to eat, and *auto*, which means self. It is, therefore, loosely translated to self-eating. In the simplest scientific terms, autophagy is a process that takes place in the eukaryotes where cytoplasmic cargo from within the vesicles is sent to the lysosome for degradation.

Autophagy and Lysosomes

[2] Eaten Alive: A History of Macroautophagy https://www.ncbi.nlm.nih.gov/pmc/articles/PMC3616322/

Christian de Duve discovered the mechanism of intracellular protein degradation. He discovered an acid phosphatase activity latency in the process of consecutive centrifugation of a rat liver homogenate. During this discovery, scientists were perplexed and unable to understand how or why a cell would consume its components. The simplest explanation for this was that perhaps, through autophagy, the cells were operating a rubbish disposal system for the body. However, further studies down the line have revealed that this process does not just get rid of old proteins, damaged organelles and toxic or invading microorganisms, but is also an adaptive automatic response to generate energy and provide nutrients whenever the body is exposed to certain stressful situations.

The study has since branched into pathophysiology, in the process indicating possibilities in the advancement of science into an immune response, neurodegeneration, cancer studies, aging, and development.

Developing the Idea of Autophagy

While not much effort has been made in tracing the origin of the membrane around the autophagosome, de Duve intimated that the sequestered membranes originate from the performed membranes, like the endoplasmic reticulum. At the cellular level, a study of rat liver cells revealed autophagy, though it was more pronounced in the livers of starved rats. It was not until 1967 that de Duve and his team discovered glucagon[3].

Building on this knowledge, Pfeifer[4] later revealed that autophagy was inhibited by insulin. Other scientists who contributed to this study include Schworer and Mortimore, whose studies showed that the end-products of autophagy, amino acids, inhibited autophagy in rat liver cells.

These findings have formed the basis of most studies into autophagy over the years, including the modern understanding of autophagy as an energy-generating and adaptive catabolic process.

Gordon and Seglen would, later on, conduct a biochemical analysis of autophagy, identifying 3-methyladenine as the pharmacological reagent that acts as an autophagy inhibitor[5]. In this study, they also produced evidence that phosphatases and protein kinases are responsible for regulating autophagy.

Between the 1950s and 1980s, most of the studies into autophagy were built around morphological analysis. Most of these studies focused on the terminal level of autophagy, and what happened before and after lysosome fusion.

---

[3] Participation of lysosomes induced autophagy in cellular autophagy induced in rat liver by glucagon https://www.ncbi.nlm.nih.gov/pubmed/6055998

[4] Inhibition by insulin of the formation of autophagic vacuoles in rat liver https://www.ncbi.nlm.nih.gov/pubmed/670291

[5] Assays to monitor autophagy progression in cell cultures https://www.ncbi.nlm.nih.gov/pmc/articles/PMC5617966/

De Duve proposed a theory that most living cells need a non-specific system for bulk segregation and portion digestion in their lysosomes for their cytoplasm. A few years later, Weibel and Bolender conducted a study proving that autophagy can engulf specific organelles. Further studies have revealed the possibility of selective autophagy, especially on higher eukaryotes and yeast.

Molecular Autophagy Control

In the 1990s, scientists delved deeper into the study of molecular autophagy. These studies were aimed at genetic manipulation of autophagy towards advancement in human health and disease.

Autophagy was initially a mammalian concern. However, studies into autophagy control were built on tractable yeast studies. The morphology of autophagy in mammals had a semblance to the morphology of autophagy in yeast. In 1997, the first autophagy-related gene, ATGI was identified and published[6]. Following this study, screening for mutant genes

[6] A novel protein kinase required for the autophagic process in Saccharomyces cerevisiae https://www.ncbi.nlm.nih.gov/pubmed/9224897

that affected unique mitophagy was carried out, and genes ATG32 and ATG33 were discovered.

While there is a similarity between macroautophagy, mitophagy, pexophagy, and the Cvt pathway, they all have unique differences. Macroautophagy is a non-selective process, while all the others are selective. Non-specific macroautophagy, mitophagy, and pexophagy are all degradative, but on the other hand, the Cvt pathway is a biosynthetic process where resident hydrolases are delivered to the vacuoles.

After the identification of the ATG genes in yeast, molecular scientists became more interested in analyzing and studying autophagy in higher eukaryotes. The first mammalian autophagy genes, ATG5 and ATG12, were discovered by Mizushima[7]. However, what would become an important discovery in the autophagy studies in higher eukaryotes was the discovery of the ATG8 homologue, MAP1LC3[8]. This would later form the basis of the current studies and findings in autophagy.

Most of the recent studies into autophagy have revealed a level of complexity especially in regulating multicellular eukaryotes. Screening of human cells revealed different components that interact with autophagy-concerned

---

[7] Transgenic rescue of ATG5-null mice from neonatal lethality with neuron-specific expression of ATG5
https://www.ncbi.nlm.nih.gov/pmc/articles/PMC5388233/

[8] Role of mammalian ATG8/LC3 family in Autophagy
https://www.ncbi.nlm.nih.gov/pmc/articles/PMC5070729/

proteins in the transduction pathways which control the process of autophagy.

While there is still a lot of disparity in the origin of the autophagosome membrane, scientists have recently suggested the possibility of autophagosome formation taking place in the plasma membrane, mitochondrial outer membrane and endoplasmic reticulum membrane.

Autophagy Regulation

An important breakthrough in the autophagy studies occurred after the rapamycin kinase was identified. The rapamycin kinase regulates protein synthesis, cell-cycle progression, and cell growth. The Meijer group in 1995 proved that rapamycin was responsible for autophagy in hepatocytes, following successful studies in rats. They also proved that rapamycin is responsible for relieving the inhibitory effect that amino acids have on autophagy.

In this study, they also proved the stimulation of the ribosomal protein S6 phosphorylation by amino acids. This process is inhibited by rapamycin and provides a connection between rapamycin kinase-dependent regulation and amino acid-dependent regulation. Though research in this field had been inconsistent and inconclusive prior, Ohsumi's lab studies provided proof that rapamycin was responsible for autophagy induction in yeast.

Through the history of studies in autophagy, three important tenets are evident. First, there is a need to dig further into the study of autophagy, especially to understand the regulatory pathways that are responsible for controlling autophagy. Special emphasis should be in understanding how different cells set the intensity and specificity of autophagy from signaling inputs.

Second, what we know about autophagy is basic information. There is so much more about this study that is yet to be unearthed. While autophagy can be construed as a protective mechanism, especially to preserve energy and nutrients when faced with starvation, or to help the body clear invasive pathogens, damaged organelles, and defective proteins, there is still so much more to be discovered.

Third, that there are a lot of questions that demand answers especially about the molecular actions of proteins, the sequestration mechanism for vesicle formation, and the reason for the specificity in selection during autophagy.

The good thing is that the knowledge of autophagy in the field of research keeps growing, and given the progress that has been made in the past, a deeper understanding of autophagy might help in fighting diseases and supporting good health.

Chapter 3: The Health Benefits

Autophagy loosely refers to *self-eating*. Autophagy is the process by which the body rids itself of damaged cells by consuming them. It is important in that it supports the creation of new, healthier cells, and is often considered a basic step in longevity and cell regeneration.

Other than creating new cells, autophagy is also a process where foreign material is destroyed. This includes bacteria, pathogens, and viruses. The body detoxifies through this process. As you grow older, autophagy slows down, and you become vulnerable to things like Parkinson's disease. However, even as you get older, there are ways of rejuvenating autophagy to prevent some of the health risks in old age before they even manifest.

Several benefits are associated with autophagy. These have been discussed at length in several scientific journals, highlighting their highs and lows, and the risks involved.

Slows Down Ageing

One of the perks of autophagy is that it helps to slow down

the aging process. Why does the body form wrinkles as a sign of old age? Aging happens because the cellular repair process is no longer as effective as it used to be while you were younger. For this reason, you experience a higher rate of accumulation of damaged components at a cellular level, which eventually translates to degeneration in your organs and tissues.

Based on several studies, aging is a genetically influenced process, and it can be affected by metabolic signaling genes. Recent studies into autophagy have further revealed that most of the genes involved in aging especially the AMP-dependent kinase (AMPK) and the nutrient sensor TOR are key autophagy regulators.

By reinvigorating the autophagy process, your body can withstand extreme conditions, especially since it gets rid of damaged macromolecules more efficiently. Autophagy, therefore, gets rid of accumulated toxic materials, in the process encouraging body maintenance at the cellular level. Therefore, this means that autophagy is important in promoting longevity by helping your body recover faster from cellular damage.

Evidence of the role that autophagy plays in slowing down the aging process has been presented in different studies, especially on yeast and multicellular organisms like flies. Studies examining Drosophila have also been successful in understanding the specificity of autophagy. These studies are aimed at the use of autophagy in therapeutic venues, and further to support the cause of autophagy in extending the lifespan of organisms.

While there is a lot to look forward to regarding the role of autophagy in the aging process, there is still so much more to be done. Scientists who have conducted studies in autophagy contend that there is more to this subject than has been discovered. It is a complex process, and one of the challenges that experts have at the moment is determining the process of selecting a membrane source for the formation of autophagosomes.

Speculatively, autophagy is a selective process. While there is evidence of the fact that it can slow down aging, concrete proof of the same is still unclear. This creates a knowledge gap that scientists are interested in filling up to completely understand the complexities behind autophagy, and how it can be used in a healthy aging process.

Prevent Cancer and Degenerative Diseases

Tumors grow and spread through genome mutation. Autophagy can suppress the growth of tumors by inhibiting the process of genome mutation. General autophagy functions include maintaining a good turnover for organelles and proteins and at the same time making sure the body maintains a homeostatic balance.

Autophagy has a damage mitigation role which is useful in fighting tumor cells. It suppresses instability in genomes, in the process limiting the progress and growth of tumors. Other than that, it can also impede the propagation of cancerous cells that have signs of malignant mutations. This is a process that encourages senescence from oncogenes. By supporting senescence, autophagy hinders the spread of oncogenic mutations, in the process slowing down the advancement of tumors.

Another way that autophagy slows down the growth and spread of tumors is by suppressing chronic inflammation. Autophagy is a homeostatic process. It gets rid of damaged cellular components and toxins from the body, while at the same time supporting the synthesis and degradation of lipids. In so doing, autophagy suppresses genome instability, slows down cellular damage, and reduces inflammation to the affected parts.

In a condition where autophagy is suppressed, there is a build-up of toxins, and this eventually causes inflammation and death to affected cells. If this happens in organs and tissues like the liver, this creates an environment where cancers can thrive.

Autophagy further offers supporting resources to aid in damage mitigation and provide a metabolic boost. Therefore, even when you are under undue stress, your body cells will still thrive. The role of autophagy, therefore, lies in inhibiting inflammation and genetic instability which often leads to the growth and spread of tumors. By stimulating autophagy, therefore, it is possible to prevent or effectively succeed in managing tumorigenesis.

Good for Your Complexion

Activating autophagy is as easy as changing or carefully monitoring your diet. Concerning your diet, you need to stay away from processed food because they limit the process of autophagy.

The biggest challenge with processed food is the oils they contain. We take in so many different types of oils, most of which are not healthy at all, but we barely realize it because we are addicted to the *eating out* culture.

When we talk about complexion, how does autophagy come into the picture? The quality of your skin deteriorates and you end up losing basic skin functions as you grow older. What the body loses in collagen can be restored through autophagy, helping you get back that glowing, plump skin complexion.

The dermis layer of the skin houses elastin and collagen, components that deteriorate over time. However, by activating autophagy, you revitalize the elastin cells and collagen, and your skin restores the elasticity you were used to when you were younger. This happens because instead of enhancing the cell turnover rate, you provide a collagen boost for your body, giving you a youthful appearance. Besides, there is a plus to this – autophagy also reduces inflammation in your skin.

Reduce Inflammation

Inflammation is the body's way of responding to tissue injury and infection. The infection causes changes in the local edema and vascular permeability. Inflammatory responses to infection are often associated with a range of disorders like inflammatory bowel disease, asthma, heart disease and so forth.

Evidence has emerged in recent years suggesting that autophagy plays an important role in helping the body clear bacteria and toxins. Other than that, autophagy also interacts with the inflammatory processes, hindering the progression of diseases.

When discussing the role of autophagy in inflammation, it is important to mention that autophagy can reduce or increase the inflammatory responses in the body. Autophagy will initiate immune responses in the aftermath of a pathogen invasion, a procedure that causes inflammation.

However, after the immune response of clearing the antigens for which the immune response was initiated, autophagy will then reduce the inflammation. It is also responsible for eliminating pro-immune response molecules that are often produced in the cells in light of a toxic invasion.

Immunity Boost

A healthy body relies on cells that are functioning well. Therefore, when we talk about boosting immunity, autophagy is a subject that is not far off. Since autophagy can help in preventing diseases, including cancer and neurodegenerative diseases, you can also look forward to boosting your immunity. In the absence of autophagy, body cells will fill up with debris and toxins, and as they die or malfunction, the body will struggle to get rid of them, which only makes your situation worse.

Perhaps the best news on this front is that optimizing autophagy for your body is not difficult. One of the most recommended ways is healthy fasting. However, you can also boost your efforts by adding healthy foods to your diet, exercise, and nutritional supplements.

Some of the threats to your immunity are so common they form a part of your daily life. These include processed foods, GMOs and EMFs. In the beginning, you might feel like autophagy is a tall order. With patience, you can manage the autophagy tasks especially by taking things step by step. While you are at it, remember not to stress your body too much. Allow yourself enough time to rest, and invest in an exercise routine that will help you boost your health.

Prolong Lifespan

By activating autophagy, your body can counteract the effect of damaged cell components, in the process improving the efficiency of cell metabolism. Autophagy is an automatic response that the body initiates when under duress, helping your body conserve energy and become more resilient at a cellular level.

In this capacity, autophagy gets rid of mitophagy (dysfunctional mitochondria) which produces toxic reactive oxygen species and hinders healthy cell growth. This process, in the long run, helps to prolong the life of different species that have been examined for the benefits of autophagy.

Autophagy is a process that keeps your system in the proper functioning mode most, if not all the time. It is regular maintenance. Anything that works towards fine-tuning your body for optimal performance will help you live longer. Through autophagy, your body can ward off opportunistic infections and diseases. The good thing about autophagy is that even if there is an infectious outbreak and it is challenging a lot of people, your body should be doing just fine. This is possible because autophagy can boost your immunity. The body works by naturally responding to changes in its environment. It will find ways to deal with toxins and prevent them from making you fall sick.

Improve Muscle Performance

In the course of exercise and other strenuous activities that you engage in from time to time, your body exerts a lot of stress on its cells. You consume a lot of energy, and in response to this and to keep you healthy while exercising, the cell components become worn out faster than when you are not exercising.

To keep the normal balance, your body initiates autophagy to respond to the demand within the cells. Autophagy will enable your cells to maintain a homeostatic balance in cellular energy consumption, reduce the amount of energy you need externally by recycling the energy molecules already available. Autophagy will also get rid of toxic cell components that might cause damage to your body before they accumulate and start causing problems.

Chapter 4: Ways to Initiate Autophagy

Autophagy is an active process that takes place in all the body cells. However, there are situations where it can be increased or slowed down. When the body is under stress, or you are going through nutrient deprivation, autophagy will increase. What this means, therefore is that you can make use of good stress mechanisms like exercise or calorie restrictions to induce autophagy. The following are some of the most effective ways of initiating autophagy:

- High-Intensity Interval Training (HIIT)
- Restorative Sleep
- Intermittent Fasting
- Protein Fasting
- Ketogenic Diet

High-Intensity Interval Training (HIIT)

If you are ever interested in changing your body composition, exercise is one of the tricks that will work for you. There are no shortcuts here, just hard work and determination. HIIT is one of the most effective alternatives that you have in this respect. A lot of the exercise routines are not as effective as they are supposed to be. You spend a lot of time on them, running aimlessly on the treadmill to no end.

The thing about HIIT is that you change the fat-to-muscle ratio. HIIT will work best when you combine it with an appropriate diet, like Intermittent Fasting. HIIT is preferable to conventional cardio when you are working towards activating autophagy.

Through HIIT, you burn more calories than through any other workout means. The good thing about HIIT is that even after you are done with the workout session, you will still be burning calories.

This happens in the period right after your exercise routine, also referred to as excess post-exercise oxygen consumption. During this period, your body is trying to restore the conditions that existed before you started working out that day. In essence what happens is that you have finished your workout routine, but your body is still consuming energy, providing additional benefits.

Experts advise that you consider at least 20 minutes of HIIT or any other rigorous activity three days of the week. HIIT workouts will help you shed up to 15% more calories as compared to other conventional workout routines, and all this is as a result of the calories that you will burn after you are through with the exercise. One of the perks of HIIT is that it is so intense, you will burn more fat in a very short time.

It is the restorative element behind HIIT that helps to propagate autophagy. Autophagy initiates a response in the body to establish a homeostatic balance. Creating this balance helps your body restore itself to a properly functioning state.

HIIT is also associated with higher performance, and an increased endurance level and speed. HIIT reduces the amount of time you spend working out because it involves your anaerobic and aerobic systems. You keep pushing yourself until you get to a point where you feel you cannot breathe anymore.

Since you go hard for about 20 minutes and call it a day through HIIT, you will be training your body to become optimally efficient. Apart from that, you will also notice results faster than any other form of exercise. Apart from inducing autophagy and the advantages that have been addressed herein, the following are some of the other benefits you will enjoy through HIIT:

- Improved sex drive
- Increased testosterone production

- Higher energy level
- Enhanced muscle tone
- Enhanced production of the fitness hormone, HGH (human growth hormone)

Restorative Sleep

Autophagy and sleep go hand in hand. When you are asleep, your body is not getting any nutrients. Therefore, the body has to find a way to make it through to the next meal (hopefully you do not eat while asleep). Autophagy is strongly linked to circadian rhythm, that controls sleep. Quality sleep is important in inducing autophagy. When you are asleep, the body has to find other ways of getting by since it is not getting fed until your next meal.

Most of the debates about how to get and maintain a healthy weight usually discuss movement and eating right, and ignore sleep altogether. More often sleep is only considered as a means of rest. More than 35% of the human population is sleep-deprived, at least according to the CDC. The real statistics on the ground could be worse, given the stressful environments that we live in.

If you are not getting enough sleep, it is very easy to undo all the good work you have done through diet and exercising. Sleep and your fat cells are correlated. After a poor night's sleep, you often wake up feeling confused, dazed and exhausted. This is not just the brain and body that is feeling grumpy, but at a cellular level, your fat cells are too. Lack of quality sleep results in metabolic grogginess.

After consecutive nights of sleep deprivation or lack of quality sleep, the hormones that control your fat cells will feel the pinch. The body is no longer able to use the insulin in your body, causing a disruption. This is not a good sign because if insulin is working as it should, your fat cells can get rid of lipids and fatty acids from the blood, preventing unnecessary hoarding. If this is not happening, the blood will be loaded with lipids, and over time excess insulin is stored in the wrong places like the liver. Thus, begins your struggle with diabetes and other associated diseases.

It gets worse, leptin and ghrelin are the hormones that control hunger. The lower the production of leptin in your fat cells, the hungrier you get. If the body is producing more ghrelin, it stimulates hunger pangs, slows down your metabolism and increases the amount of fat the body stores. Therefore, for optimal weight loss, your body needs to balance the production of leptin and ghrelin, yet all this is impeded by poor or no sleep at all.

Intermittent Fasting

One of the profound benefits of intermittent fasting (IF will be discussed in detail later on) is that it supports autophagy, breaking down and recycling damaged cellular organelles and molecules. When you are properly fed, insulin is increased, and the rate of autophagy in your body is at an all-time low. However, when you are hungry, the reverse happens. The rate of autophagy can increase up to five times.

Most of the benefits of intermittent fasting and calorie restriction are associated with an increase in autophagy. When you fast often, you effectively reset the rate of autophagy, and your body operates at the level of a much younger person. All this happens because insulin has been reduced.

Alongside intermittent fasting, you also need to consider exercises. Exercise is important in that it improves your sensitivity to insulin. Therefore, if you are fasting and in shape, your insulin levels drop faster, and the process of lipolysis starts faster than someone who has not been working out. Take note that insulin resistance suppresses the function of autophagy. This is a possible explanation behind the effects of obesity and diabetes.

There are so many ways of practicing intermittent fasting. Most people consider consuming all the necessary calories during the 8-hour work period and skipping breakfast.

Everyone has a schedule that works well for them. It is advisable that you find yours and stick to it. You can try a few experiments before you find one that is ideal for you.

Nutrient deprivation is one of the fastest ways of inducing autophagy. There are different ways of going about this. A popular option is the 5:2 rule. This means that you fast for two days, but maintain a normal eating plan for the other five days of the week. The body, during this period, breaks down proteins, and in the process gets rid of toxins that might be present in the body at the time. When you practice this diet, be keen not to cheat on your fasting days.

Protein Fasting

Protein fasting is a process where you cycle between a period of normal high protein consumption and a period of low protein consumption. The effect on the body is similar to what you experience when you are fasting. You are effectively creating a protein deficiency in the body, which lowers the level of insulin. In response, the body produces more glucagon and induces autophagy. What the body is doing at this time, is to avoid storing all the foods you are consuming as fat, but instead burn fat and build muscle.

One of the reasons why a protein fast is successful is because the body is unable to produce the protein it needs. The body, therefore, needs to find a way of recycling the proteins that you have consumed. Should there be a deficiency in the protein intake, autophagy kicks in, instructing the body to initiate a recycling process, and takes it a notch higher.

During the protein cycle, the body has room to recycle any of the old proteins that might still be lingering in the body. These are the ones that eventually cause inflammation. As this process is going on, the body also goes into maintenance mode, cleaning out its cells without necessarily causing muscle loss in the process. Therefore, this is a good way of getting that lean body you have always desired. The body binds to toxins that are present in the cytoplasm and moves them out of the cell environment. Protein fasting works in the same way that fasting does, by reducing the mechanistic target of rapamycin (mTOR) and insulin levels in the body. These are responsible for metabolism and cellular growth.

By periodically reducing the level of mTOR and increasing them a short while later after eating, the body has enough room to repair and rebuild its cells, helping you build a leaner body. This is also responsible for controlling aging and the spread of disorders like diabetes, cancer and heart disease.

However, while protein fasting is a good thing, remember that you should not do it every other day. A body that is protein deficient daily can suffer in the long run. This is why a 5:2 intermittent fasting cycle is recommended, allowing the body enough room to replenish its protein resources. Alternatively, you can adopt a ketogenic diet.

Ketogenic Diet

Ketosis is one of the easiest ways of inducing the body cells to clean up. A low carbohydrate diet (less than 50 grams of carbs) induces the liver to produce ketones. Ketones are a fuel source for the brain and the body especially when you are not getting the carbohydrates you need. They provide readily available and usable sources of energy. Ketones are also responsible for anti-aging and protecting the body from brain damage.

Ketones trigger the body cells to clean up in the same way that fasting does. They activate lysosomes to break down residual proteins that are either damaged or old. It is like green energy, for the body. The good thing about it is that you reap the benefits of fasting, without actually fasting.

In the process of protein breakdown, the body naturally targets non-essential proteins first, especially proteins from junk food. The good thing about this diet is that given the amount of protein that you consume, the body can use the food you eat to produce ketones and glucose it needs without having to break down lean muscle for survival.

The ketogenic diet, a high fat, low carb diet, is a good way to induce autophagy and reduce your protein consumption. When you consume too many proteins than the body needs, the excess is converted into sugar. This does not happen to fat, however. A ketogenic diet, therefore, trains the body to change the source of fuel to ketones.

Therefore, getting your body into ketosis is one of the easiest ways of activating autophagy. Besides, when you reduce your intake of proteins and carbs, you are simply keeping away toxins from the body. The body has fewer obstacles to power through, and your autophagy operates at the highest level.

Chapter 5: Water Fasting

Water fasting is a fasting method where you are restricted from consuming anything other than water. In recent years, it has become a very popular mechanism for weight loss. Several benefits have been attributed to water fasting, including the ability to lower the risk of infection, chronic diseases, and activating autophagy.

There still exists limited research on water fasting, so it is important to do it with a lot of caution. There are health risks that might be involved, so it is not a suitable option for everyone. People often consider water fasting for different reasons, including the following:

- Preparation for a medical procedure
- Detoxing
- Weight loss
- Spiritual or religious reasons
- For the health benefits

Given that most of the limited studies in water fasting have highlighted health benefits and the possibility of a reduced risk of diabetes, heart disease, and cancer, a lot of people are increasingly interested in water fasting.

Benefits of Water Fasting

Water fasting is linked to several benefits, both in animal and human studies. In the quest to lose weight, a lot of people are torn between different dietary procedures. The choice between juice cleansing and water fasting is one that most people struggle to make. While water fasting demands that you only consume water, juice fasting allows you to include vegetables and fruits in a juiced form, providing you with antioxidants, minerals, vitamins, and calories.

While juice fasting has its benefits, it is important to mention that this is a diet that lacks a lot of important nutrients. Therefore, in the long run, you might still add weight after fasting, because your body will struggle to readjust itself to its normal metabolic rate.

The following are some of the reasons why you might want to think about water fasting:

Promotes Autophagy

Autophagy is a process where the old cell components are recycled and broken down. Studies into autophagy have revealed that it can help in managing and protecting you from diseases like heart disease and cancer.

Through autophagy, the damaged cell components are unable to accumulate in the body, creating free radicals that eventually cause cancer. This is one of the ways of preventing the growth of cancer cells.

Studies in animals have shown how important water fasting is to supporting autophagy. It does not end there either, and these studies also prove that it is possible to prolong your life through autophagy

Reduce Risk of Chronic Diseases

There is proof that water fasting can reduce your risk exposure to diseases like heart disease, cancer, and diabetes. A study observed 30 healthy adults who were water fasting for a day. After this exercise, their blood triglyceride and cholesterol levels had reduced. These are two of the risk factors responsible for heart disease.

Some animal studies into water fasting revealed that it could also help in protecting the heart from damage through free radicals. These are unstable molecules that often cause damage to cells, and are active in the propagation of chronic diseases. Water fasting also hinders the growth of genes that support the growth of cancer cells, thereby improving the impact that chemotherapy has on patients.

Reduce Blood Pressure

If you are struggling with blood pressure, you should consider supervised water fasting, as it has been proven to improve symptoms. A study of 68 people after 14 days on supervised water fasting revealed more than 80% of the patients had their blood pressure drop to a healthy level.

Most of the studies that have been conducted lasted a longer time than the average water fasting period. These studies last a few days. Therefore, even with their success rate being so impressive, it is still a challenge addressing the link to short-term water fasting that lasts between 24 and 72 hours, and the impact on blood pressure.

Improve Leptin and Insulin Sensitivity

Cellular metabolism is controlled by insulin and leptin. Leptin helps the body by making you feel full, while insulin draws nutrients from the bloodstream. Through water fasting, you tweak the body in such a way that it becomes more sensitive to the presence of insulin and leptin. Heightened sensitivity helps to make your hormones more effective. You are able to reduce blood sugar faster in case you have an insulin-sensitive body. Leptin sensitivity is a good thing because your body can process hunger signals more efficiently, reducing the risk of obesity.

Forget About Cravings and Hunger

If you are getting on the water fasting diet, you might struggle during the first phase, but over time as you get used to it, the hunger and cravings disappear. It is not just about them disappearing, they also become easier to manage. Once you get used to the fasting program, it makes it easier for you to deal with hunger down the line. The water fasting diet is easier to manage compared to a lot of diets that are not as restrictive as this is.

By managing your cravings and hunger, you are in a better position to maintain your weight loss goals even after you have achieved your desired weight. Most people struggle to keep their weight after they are through with the diet they are on and add back weight soon after. Some people add more weight, leaving them in a worse situation than they were before they started working out.

Safe Water Fasting

How long you can water fast depends on whether you are new to this, or if you have been doing it for a while. For beginners, do not push yourself more than 72 hours or three days. These are the basics. Even for those who have some experience with water fasting, three days is enough.

If you feel you need to go further than that, it is advisable that you seek medical supervision, and probably seek admission into a fasting retreat. Why would you consider a fasting retreat? This is a good place for you because it creates an enabling environment for you to see through the fast. A retreat is a safe place because it takes away temptations and distractions. Apart from that, you are around people who share a common goal, fasting. Retreats are also a good idea because you have an expert who will address your concerns as, and when they arise.

Water Fasting for Weight Loss

A lot of people these days consider water fasting as a means of losing weight. This is one of the safest options available. Individuals who have tried water fasting for weight loss have reported losing up to 3 pounds a day. However, you must realize that these are dependent on reasons and features that are unique to different people, depending on their body physiology.

How much weight you lose after completing a water fast depends on how long you are on the fast, and your body. What you will lose when you start is water weight. The actual fat burning does not happen at least until after one or two days.

It is possible to lose up to a pound of weight a day on the water fast diet. However, in case your diet has been composed mostly of processed foods, your body retains a lot of sodium and water. Therefore, at the beginning of your water fast, you can lose even up to three pounds each day. As you gradually fast over time, your body will create a balance and lose roughly half a pound a day.

Preparing for a Water Fast

Having decided that you are starting a water fast, you must be adequately prepared for what lies ahead. Other than losing weight, you must also realize that water fasting is an extreme detox process. In case you have never tired detoxing in your life, you must be very careful about how you go about this.

There might be severe reactions if you do not do it well. In the most intensive phase of the detox, usually within the first three days, some of the reactions you might experience include vomiting, nausea, headaches, diarrhea, migraines, and dizziness. Your body will also hurt a lot.

To reduce the effect of these reactions, you should consider preparing adequately for this diet. Here is a guideline that will make things relatively more manageable for you:

Organic Foods – Consider switching to organic foods. There are a lot of pesticides that find their way into your food, and consuming non-organic food will see you consume toxins from the pesticides.

Eating Meat – It is time you stopped eating meat. This might not go down well with a lot of people, but meat is one of the weakest sources of proteins, not mentioning the toxins and hormones that are present in the animal.

While ditching meat from your diet, consider foods that are rich in amino acids like seeds, vegetables, and fruits.

Coffee – Stop drinking coffee and other caffeinated drinks. If it is difficult for you to quit this instantly, wean yourself off caffeine slowly. This is important as it will help you restore your adrenal glands, and at the same time protect you from struggling with coffee withdrawal.

Alcohol – While we are on the subject of quitting caffeine, do away with alcohol too. Quitting alcohol allows the liver to use the glutathione for detox instead of metabolizing alcohol.

Gluten – You must avoid eating dairy and gluten as these are allergenic and produce mucus, which is difficult for most people to digest.

Fruits – If you have not been eating fruits, this is the time for you to consider taking them up. Where possible, eat three servings of berries a day. Berries offer antioxidant support which will be useful for you when you are on a detox meal plan.

Colon Cleansing

Before you start a water fast, you must perform a colon cleanse. If you do not do it before you start, perform a colon cleanse after fasting for a few days. The idea here is to get rid of stools that remain in the digestive tract for a long time, and the bacteria that remain in the colon and starts producing toxins.

Why is a colon cleanse important? The toxins that have been mentioned might be absorbed into the bloodstream in the course of a water fast, poisoning your body in the process.

How much water should you drink?

When you are on a water fast, how much water is safe for you to drink? Ladies are advised to drink around 11 cups of water a day, which is equivalent to 2.5 liters, compared to 13 cups a day for men, which is equivalent to 3 liters of water.

Most people struggle to keep the recommended water limits. A workaround for this would be filling water bottles in the morning. Keep these in plain sight, where you can see them, and have them act as a reminder that you should be drinking some water. Space out your water drinking sessions through the day. You would not want to drink too much water at a go.

Transitioning from a Water Fast

While you are on the water fast, you will not be eating any food, just water. Therefore, your digestive system might not be ready for you to take an immediate dive into solid food or a normal diet almost immediately. If you force yourself into eating foods that are not easy to digest, you might end up spending most of your time post-fasting, in a hospital.

There are some recommended foods that you can start eating when you complete your water fast without any complications. These are as follows:

- Vegetable juices
- Fruit juices
- Yogurt
- Raw fruits
- Leafy green raw vegetables like spinach
- Cooked vegetables

- Eggs
- Dairy
- Vegetable soup
- Meat and fish

Start with the soft, liquid and easy to digest foods when you break your fast, and gradually work your way to things like meat and fish. When you are comfortable with hard food, you can then get back to eating everything else.

Tips for Surviving a Water Fast

Water fasting, like any other form of fasting, is not a walk in the park. Many have tried and given up along the way. Water fasting might take a toll on you. However, if you are adequately prepared, nothing should scare you. Here are some useful tips that will help you get through a water fast:

Watch what you drink

A water fast is an important part of your life. You, therefore, need to make sure you are using quality water. If you are planning to start a water fast, do not use tap water. There is a lot of garbage and toxins in tap water. Consider getting spring water as you prepare for your fast. Where possible, find someone who can deliver it to your home.

Avoid Industrial products

During the fasting period, try and stay away from products like creams, body oils, and shampoo. The body absorbs such items into the bloodstream. Where possible, do not use toothpaste. Instead, you can brush your teeth with plain water, and use a tongue scraper.

Only water allowed

This is a serious factor that some people never take seriously. When you start a water fast, have it at the back of your mind that only water is allowed. This means that you will not be having any coffee, lemons, vitamins, supplements or tea.

Get your mind in the game

Fasting is as much a mental concern as it is about keeping away from food. You need something to keep your mind occupied, otherwise the hunger pangs might drive you crazy. This is the time for you to invest in some motivational or inspirational books, podcasts or playlists. You can even create an entire playlist of movies or TV shows that you can watch during this time to get your mind at ease.

Concerning motivation, you can also consider speaking to a friend or family member who will help you get through the fast. When you have someone supporting you, it can be much easier for you to get through a water fast. Having someone around is good because you motivate, encourage and accompany one another when things are difficult.

Quality rest

Allow yourself enough time to rest as much as you can. Physically, when you are fasting, you are not supposed to engage in strenuous activities. It doesn't matter how strong you feel you are, and this is not the time for you to be exerting yourself. However, on the first day, you can consider an intense workout. This is aimed at pushing the body to maximize the use of its utility supplies.

Have a Purpose

Having a reason for fasting should be one of the first things you think about when you start fasting. Do not go about it blindly. Your reason for fasting is what will help you keep working hard to meet your goals. This is what motivates you whenever you feel you are unable to proceed. It is a constant reminder that you are in this for the long haul.

Chapter 6: Other Types of Fasting and Diets

Intermittent Fasting

Intermittent Fasting, popularly abbreviated as IF, is a popular mode of fasting today. Take note that for thousands of years people have been fasting in different unique cultures all over the world. So, what makes IF different from all this? IF proponents suggest this as a more comfortable, sustainable and convenient way to lose weight while at the same time improving your health in general.

IF is about limiting the consumption of beverages and foods that are calorie-rich to a specific time during the day, and for the rest of the day, you stay without food. To clear this up a bit, you limit consumption to 8 hours and stay 16 hours without food. This is why at times it is also referred to as the 16/8 Intermittent Fasting Diet.

This diet is convenient in that you are free to perform it as you wish, either daily, or on specific days of the week according to your preference. IF has become popular especially with people who want to burn fat and lose weight.

Many diets have a strict set of regulations, which is one of the most significant differences between IF and all the rest. On this diet, you can achieve the expected or desired results with minimum effort, and less strain on yourself.

This is one of the most flexible diets and should fit most lifestyles comfortably. Other than weight loss, IF has also been recommended in the past for individuals who want to boost their brain function, improve control of blood sugar, and live a longer, healthier life.

How Does It Work?

IF initiates physiological changes in the body at the most basic level, the cellular level. This diet is useful in that it can help you improve your insulin sensitivity, with burning fat and optimizing blood sugar levels.

IF also increases the level of the HGH – human growth hormone, which helps in cell regeneration. HGH is also responsible for decreased body fat and enhanced body composition.

IF is also touted as a good way of inducing autophagy. Through autophagy, your body gets rid of toxins and waste, enhancing cellular repair in the process. In the recent past, some studies[9] have suggested that IF can also protect the body from brain aging and chronic diseases by manipulating molecules and genes in the body.

Starting the Diet

Choose an 8-hour window within which you can participate in this program, and ensure your food intake is limited. For most busy people, an ideal program starts at noon and ends at around 8 or 9 p.m. In this window, you can skip breakfast and spend most of the fasting period asleep, but still manage to squeeze in a few snacks during the day, and a well-balanced meal at lunch and dinner.

Another possible schedule would be from 9 a.m. because it allows you to enjoy a sumptuous, healthy breakfast, a healthy lunch meal at your normal lunch hour and a snack later in the afternoon, or an early, light dinner, then fast through the night, with most of the evening spent asleep.

Before you settle on the ideal pattern, try out a few experiments and settle on something that suits your schedule. While this plan is about fasting, you also need to keep your hunger in check. Therefore, during the hours when you are not fasting, it would be wise to have some snacks or small meals spaced evenly.

To realize improved results fast enough, you should consider

---

[9] Caloric restriction and intermittent fasting: Two potential diets for successful brain aging https://www.ncbi.nlm.nih.gov/pmc/articles/PMC2622429/#S2title

including only healthy foods packed with nutrients in this diet plan. You need to have lots of fruits, vegetables, whole grains, healthy fats, and protein-rich foods. In terms of the beverage selection, consider unsweetened coffee or tea, and water, because apart from helping you hydrate, they also manage your appetite.

Benefits of Intermittent Fasting

One of the reasons why this is a popular diet is because of how easy it is to follow, and the fact that it is sustainable in the long run. The time normally spent preparing food can instead be devoted to other productive uses. The following are some of the benefits of starting an IF diet:

Longevity – There is not much practical evidence in humans, but lab results from animal studies indicate the prospect of extended longevity on this diet.

Improved brain function – One of the perks of starting the IF diet is that it induces the brain to regenerate new nerve cells which eventually improve your cognitive faculty.

Control blood sugar – On this diet, you can reduce insulin levels by around 30%. If you have been struggling with blood sugar levels, you can enjoy up to a 6% reduction, which also lowers your risk of getting diabetes.

Weight loss – By limiting your meals to just a few hours a day, you will burn calories, in the process boosting your body's metabolism, helping you lose weight.

Extended Water Fasting

Other than hydration and quenching your thirst, water can also be a useful way to lose weight. Water fasting is a form of fasting where you do not eat food but only drink water.

Even as you begin this routine, it is important that you understand the best time to go about fasting is when your body does not need a lot of energy. People often embark on water fasting for a variety of reasons, ranging from medical, personal diet reasons or even spiritual concerns.

While there is no set duration within which you can water fast, experts recommend no more than three days as the maximum time you should go without eating. You can, however, embark on a water fast for 24 hours safely.

Benefits of Water Fasting

One of the reasons why water fasting is an amazing choice is that people can benefit from it, even if they are struggling with diseases that might make it difficult for them to participate in some of the more conventional diets. Other than being overweight, some of these diseases or conditions include diabetes, high cholesterol, high blood pressure, and heart disease.

Most of the risks mentioned here are linked in a way. The body has to burn fat to generate energy when it is not getting sufficient carbohydrates. Therefore, fasting can help you lose weight as the body burns fat to produce energy.

Even as you are going about your diet, remember that you still need to find time in your schedule to exercise. To support progress in your diet, reduce your intake of sugary foods where possible.

Safe Water Fasting

Before you consider water fasting, always consult a doctor or an expert. Fasting might yield success for a lot of people, but it is not always the best option for everyone. If you fast for a long time, there are health risks that you might encounter.

Some people are not supposed to fast, or if they do, they are not supposed to keep it up for a long time. This applies to people who are either old or sick. If you have to fast under any of these circumstances, make sure you do it under supervision.

While water fasting is generally safe, it is not advisable for anyone who is underweight, under the age of 18, or older adults. Water fasting is also not recommended for people with eating disorders, breastfeeding or pregnant mothers, anyone with persistent migraines, type 1 diabetes, heart problems or if you are having a blood transfusion. You should also consult your doctor in case you are taking any medication.

If you have never fasted before, take it slow. Start your fast in a comfortable place, like at home. An ideal fast is best when you are resting. You must also be mentally prepared for a water fast, given that fasting can be emotionally and physically draining.

Keto diet

The ketogenic diet is a low-carb diet. If you follow this diet keenly, you can burn excess fat and get your desired body shape. Other than weight loss, the ketogenic diet can also offer other amazing benefits. The ketogenic diet can help you boost your performance and improve your health. One of the best things about this diet is that you can stay on it while eating normal foods. On this diet, you might not even have to concern yourself with going out of your way to find foods that are not within your budget range.
The ketogenic diet works on the principle that the body has to produce its fuel (ketones) which powers the body in the event of a shortage of glucose in the blood.

If you constantly maintain a diet that is low in carbs, the

body has to produce ketones. The body converts fat into ketones in the liver. When you start this diet, your body will be fueling its needs by burning fat. Your insulin levels drop and the rate of fat burning increases. For someone who is out to lose weight, this is a good thing.

Other than losing weight, you will also be more energetic when you are on this diet. This diet can also help you become more focused on what you are working on, or your life goals. Like most diets, you should have a reason for starting it, as this gives you purpose.

Ketosis is a metabolic state associated with the ketogenic diet, where the body produces ketones. The easiest way of inducing ketosis is through fasting. However, you cannot be fasting every single day of the year. So, if you plan on getting into ketosis through fasting, you might need to rethink your strategy. On the ketogenic diet, however, you enjoy the perks of fasting, especially weight loss, without necessarily having to go all-out fasting.

While the ketogenic diet has its benefits, some individuals should avoid it altogether. If you are breastfeeding, are taking medicine for high blood pressure or diabetes, the ketogenic diet is not for you. Get in touch with your doctor about your best course of action in terms of getting similar benefits.

Benefits of the Keto Diet

Everyone has a reason why they are on a specific diet. For the ketogenic diet, the following are some of the benefits you can look forward to enjoying:

- **Weight Loss**

Of course, most people who start the ketogenic diet want to burn as much fat as possible, so that they get the desired body shape and size. In the recent past, experts have proven that the ketogenic diet is more effective compared to most diets in weight loss and management.

- **Epilepsy Therapy**

This diet has been used effectively in managing epilepsy ever since the 1920s. It is a treatment plan that has worked for children, though in recent years scientists have started using it to manage epilepsy in adults. Individuals who are on the ketogenic diet can use fewer drugs for epilepsy, or stop taking them altogether, depending on how their body responds to the diet.

- **Endurance**

The ketogenic diet can help you improve your physical endurance level. This is because you can access the energy stashed away in your body's fat stores. The body stores energy in the form of glycogen and this can run out very fast when you are exercising. However, fat stores can store energy for weeks on end.

- **Stomach Upsets**

You will be eating healthy meals, which will help you calm your stomach. You won't have to worry about cramping, pain, and gas, and this diet can drastically improve your symptoms if you have IBS. Some people have reported noticing improvements in as little as a day.

- **Mental Calm**

A lot of people struggle with sugar swings. However, when you are on the ketogenic diet, it helps your brain maintain a steady ketone supply. As a result, you focus better, concentrate, and for people who have had issues with brain fog, the new sense of mental clarity is always a welcome change.

- **Improved Health**

The ketogenic diet among other low-carb diets is often linked to improved health markers especially for high-risk conditions like heart disease. Your insulin levels should improve, as will your blood pressure and cholesterol profile.

- **Blood Sugar Control**

If you have type-2 diabetes, this diet can help you keep your blood sugar levels in check. Some people have completely reversed type-2 diabetes by following this diet. This is possible because the ketogenic diet lowers your level of blood sugar, so you no longer need as much medication as you normally do, in the process minimizing the impact of having a high level of insulin.

- **Manage Appetite**

This diet is a good way to keep your appetite in check. It is easy to do this because when you get used to the ketogenic diet, you get used to eating only when you are hungry, and not when you feel like it. If you plan on starting an intermittent fasting diet, the ketogenic diet would be a good place to begin.

- **General Benefits**

Other than these advantages, there are some that are not so common but have been experienced by people who were on the ketogenic diet. These include normalized blood pressure, reduced migraine incidences, improve acne, reduced sugar cravings, fewer heartburn cases and reversed polycystic ovary syndrome (PCOS).

Fast Mimicking

Fast mimicking is a modified way of fasting. While a normal fasting routine would have you not eating at all, on this diet you will eat small amounts of food, but in a manner that gives you the benefits of traditional fasting.

Fast mimicking should not take more than five days. It is a diet where you will consume very few carbs, calories, and protein, but high amounts of fat. You will try to limit your calorie intake to 40% of your usual intake. In so doing, your body will remain nourished with electrolytes and nutrients, earning you the benefits of a normal fast, without the strain that comes with it.

Fast mimicking diet is more effective and safer than long-term fasting or long-term calorie restriction. The fast mimicking diet allows you the same benefits you would receive from any other diet. You reduce your calorie intake in a way that tricks the body into a fasting state. The body then has to convert stored fat into energy.

Safe Fast Mimicking

According to experts, you can look forward to the best results when your glucose ketone index is under 1.0, or after around five days. Therefore, an ideal duration for this diet is 3 – 7 days. To get the best results from this diet, you need to perform it at least once a month. However, two times a year would also be good.

It is advisable that you take measurements for different metrics before, during and after fasting. These include weight changes, ketones, and blood glucose levels. Fasting works well when you have an active environment that is rooting for you or supporting your effort. Make sure you inform those around you, not just about what you are doing, but your reasons for going on the fast mimicking diet.

During this period, do not buy foods or snacks that might interrupt your progress. If there are some in the house, get rid of them. Since your body will be more exhausted than it usually is, make sure you have a good resting plan.

Include some physical activity in your daily schedule. However, ensure you only perform light activities, and avoid strenuous exercises at this time.

Basic fast mimicking will see you consume more calories at the beginning, almost half of the total intake. Over time this should reduce to around 30% of your total caloric intake. You should try and ensure the food you consume is available in small amounts, and easily digestible.

On this diet, you do not necessarily need to have a pre-packaged box, especially for someone who needs to keep the diet low on carbs. Use the calorie percentages to guide how you space your meals through the day. It is wise to plan for all the food in your diet plan so that you have nothing to worry about.

You can have a cup of tea or coffee a day, as long as they do not have any sugars or added cream. If you have any health concerns, get in touch with your doctor before you start this diet. You might also need to supplement this diet if you want to get all the necessary electrolytes and nutrients. Some of the supplements you can use include:

- Grass-fed liver tablets for micronutrients
- Salt and magnesium for water loss
- BCAAs
- Cod liver oil
- Algal oil

The fast mimicking diet is highly recommended in case you are on a ketogenic diet. This diet allows your body to reach ketosis faster, and since you will be eating keto foods, you can have your body in ketosis throughout the diet.

24h Fast

The 24-hour fast is a form of Intermittent Fasting. You can do it once or twice a week. It is common among fitness experts. It is very straightforward. If you start it at 8 pm today, it ends at 8 pm tomorrow. You can also choose to have it timed by your meals, like breakfast to breakfast and so forth. The idea is to make sure it ends at the same time it started the previous day.

When you are on this diet, you are allowed to indulge in non-caloric beverages, coffee or water. The only thing you have to avoid is solid food. Depending on your reason for being on this diet, on your normal eating days, you should ensure you eat proper meals.

Given that most people find it difficult to go a complete 24 hours without eating, it is advisable that you practice this diet in shorter bouts, like 14 hours for a start, then work your way up to 24. It is one of those diets that demands insane discipline for you to see it through.

Chapter 7: Weight Loss

Having looked at how autophagy works, we can now have a look at how you can lose weight through autophagy. Autophagy is a powerful tool that you can harness and attain the weight you have always dreamt of. To do this, you must practice intermittent fasting. This means you will need to plan your diet in such a way that you only eat during a pre-determined time.

For the rest of the day when you are not eating, the body uses its internal energy resources to burn fat. Have you ever wondered how celebrities manage to slim down into shape for a specific role so fast? Most of them follow such a routine.

Most of the time, these individuals maintain a diet rich in protein for 1/3 of their day and fast for the other 2/3. When they are fasting, cellular metabolism takes care of the weight loss, burning fat stored from the food they had eaten earlier. Autophagy is not just good for weight loss, and there are other benefits that you will enjoy along the way, including better hair quality, skin tone and a shot at a longer lifespan.

Before jumping into autophagy to enjoy some of the benefits yourself, you must consult an expert. Talk to your doctor, nutritionist or any other expert you know. Discuss what is at stake, and how you plan to go about this. For a start you will need help spacing out your meals, considering your normal meal hours and work schedule. If you are working out, this is even more important. Everything needs to check out, or you will have a difficult time on this plan. Besides, without a good plan, you might end up wasting muscle in the process.

You also have to drink sufficient amount of water to help your body get rid of toxins that accumulate over the course of autophagy. Apart from that, hydration is important for a healthy life.

People are different, so you should not expect to replicate the results that someone else had. In your struggle to lose weight this is a mistake that most people make when they start working out, dieting or planning their lives around autophagy. In terms of the amount of weight you can lose, it depends on your body physiology.

What is more important is for you to understand what you are working towards, note the small milestones you are making and stay focused on your goals. Whether you are losing a pound a day or three, be sure to appreciate the progress you are making. This is the best way for you to stay on course, and keep yourself motivated.

Keeping Lost Weight Off

Why do you struggle to maintain weight loss after a while?

Many people have struggled with this question in the past. There are a lot of things conspiring to work against you after you hit your target weight. Most people attain their desired weight and dive back into high-calorie foods. It becomes so easy to gain weight after that.

Soon after losing weight, your body's metabolism is lower than ever. Therefore, you are burning fewer calories than you should, even when you are resting or asleep. What happens here is that your brain detects you are running low on fat supplies and signals the muscles to be minimal in consumption.

After losing weight, your body goes through a lot of changes. Your appetite will change, and more often you tend to eat more to feel satisfied. The parts of the brain that used to resist eating and make you feel satiated faster are slower. This makes it easier for you to start gaining what you lost. Coupled with the fact that your preference for high-calorie foods is at an all-time high, it is very easy to gain weight. How do you fight this?

One of the key pillars of your weight loss plan is your diet. On the other hand, if you are looking to maintain your weight loss, you should exercise more often. According to studies from the National Weight Control Registry, those who lose and keep the weight off exercise more than most average people.

These people spend at least an hour walking each day. You can also consider roughly one hour of moderate exercises. In case you engage in strenuous activities like contact sports, your exercise routine can be no more than half an hour a day.

Starting an exercise routine after losing weight can be difficult. Considering the challenges you might experience, a good idea would be to start working out while you are still losing weight. By the time you attain your desired weight, you are already used to working out, and maintenance can be more comfortable.

Other than exercise, the following are some of the other tips that will help you maintain your new weight:

- Eat a healthy breakfast every day
- Check your weight regularly
- Ensure you eat sufficient proteins to feel full, and to manage your appetite
- Monitor your carb intake
- Try to manage your stress levels
- Add vegetables and fruits to your meal plan
- Understand that you might stumble along the way
- Drink water as recommended
- Make sure you get sufficient sleep

Exercise is important in keeping weight off because it prevents the body from getting used to the metabolic slowdown that happens soon after you lose weight. Exercise will, therefore, help your body keep burning calories even when you are resting.

Besides, if you are very active, this means that you will not necessarily have to be strict with your diet as you were when you were trying to lose weight in the first place. Even if this is the case, do not just go about eating everything that you come across. Try to eat just enough calories that your body can burn.

Chapter 8: Maintaining Muscle Mass

Most people believe that the loss of muscle mass is one of the side effects of fasting. This has been the subject of several discussions and conspiracy theories about fasting. What you need to realize, however, is that when you fast properly and follow the autophagy guidelines, your muscle mass will not waste away.

The concept behind autophagy is to break something down then build it up afresh. This breakdown is the same thing that takes place in the body when you are working out at the gym. You push your muscles as far as possible, exerting stress on them. This process involves muscle damage, but after that, the body repairs the muscles, and they are regenerated, stronger and more agile than before.

Anyone who has ever spent time training will understand how this works. What you might not understand, perhaps, is how important nutrition is to the process of breaking down and building up your body, especially at the cell level.

Role of Autophagy in Maintaining Muscle Mass

Through autophagy, the body degrades defective and damaged proteins, cell membranes and organelles. The body monitors, identifies, and discards any parts of the cell that are either useless or malfunctioning. Autophagy is the clean-up process that takes place before repair and growth can be initiated.

Ejecting waste cell components is important because without this process you might experience side-effects like inappropriate muscle mass as a result of malfunctioning mitochondria accumulating in the cells.

Fasting is important in the autophagy process. When you are fasting, the body gets a signal to initiate autophagy. Therefore, when you start eating, your body automatically turns off autophagy. Even cheating on your fast with a light meal is enough to slow down the process of autophagy.

Autophagy plays an important role in maintaining muscle mass. Inhibiting or altering autophagy, therefore, can result in the degeneration of individual muscle fibers, which is associated with weak muscles in the case of unique muscle disorders. For proper muscle health, reduced and excess autophagy levels confer a detrimental effect. Excess autophagy will cause muscle loss, while reduced autophagy causes weakness from the degeneration of skeletal fiber.

What this means is that it is dangerous for you to be fasting all the time. However, you need to find the right balance for autophagy and a normally functioning body. Breaking you down and building you up is not just a function of the workout regime you are on. It is something that can also happen as a result of the diet you keep.

Autophagy Inhibition and Muscle Loss

What role does autophagy play in conditions where muscle wasting is evident? Inhibiting autophagy does not stop muscle loss or the activation of denervated muscles through atrophy. Studies have revealed that animals that experience deficient autophagy suffer more muscle loss than the ones that do not.

What is evident from studies thus far is that autophagy plays an important role in controlling muscle mass. Without autophagy, the organelle suffers, and there is an accumulation of dilated sarcoplasmic reticulum and atypical mitochondria. To be clear, having damaged cell components in the body does not have a detrimental effect on cellular function.

Muscle weakness and atrophy is caused by the presence of atypical organelles, which initiate catabolic pathways. What is important at this juncture is to control mitochondrial function.

Maintaining the Balance

Autophagy is responsible for maintaining and cleaning the body at a cellular level when you are fasting. You need to support this with proper, healthy meal plans that encourage growth. This is a good way to establish a balance in the process of muscle building, which also prevents muscle loss as you grow older.

You need to establish a balance, given that it is not wise to overeat all the time under the guise that you will fast and undo the damage. The repercussions of doing this will be dire. Create a balance where you get sufficient rest, while at the same time eating a good, healthy diet and spending a sufficient amount of time fasting too. A good balance should also be time-checked. This gives the body sufficient time to process and break down the malfunctioning cell components, and build new, stronger, healthier and bigger muscles.

Chapter 9: Closing Thoughts

In more ways than one, autophagy delves into the traditional diet and health tips that you might have come across from time to time. This book highlights autophagy in different respects that you can easily relate to. One of the challenges that most people have when they come across material like these is that they are written in such a manner that it is impossible for them to comprehend, especially the technical terms.

In the society we live in today, hunger is ostracized, treated as something that we need to shun. However, from an autophagy perspective, this is not the case. Going hungry might be the one thing that saves your life, and keeps you alive for a very long time, living a healthy life while at it.

Take note that while autophagy encourages you to go hungry from time to time, you do not have to do it all the time. In all honesty, you cannot go hungry every single day of the month, if you want to live long. Fasting, when done properly, can promote your well-being and keep you healthy. It will also help you lose weight.

The process of autophagy is important in many aspects of your life. The fact that it is an automatic process further makes your life easier. You do not have to worry about autophagy because it takes place whether you like it or not. However, what you can do is make a few changes in your life that will initiate autophagy.

The body is a system that takes care of itself. It was built that way. Your body regulates itself, detoxifies and finds a way to get by even without your input. What you can do, however, is to make things relatively easier for your body, by taking steps to initiate autophagy. On the contrary, initiating autophagy is not a difficult process.

You can learn about simple changes you can make as you go about your day, like exercising, eating right, being more active and so forth. These are the small changes that push the body and induce autophagy. For a system that is already working well, fine-tuning your body will make your systems more efficient, and you will live a longer, more productive life.

Regarding the health benefits associated with autophagy, there is so much more that we can look forward to. Currently, autophagy has taken center stage in revolutionary research studies in the management and treatment of cancer. Autophagy is also being used in managing epilepsy, not just in children, but in adults too. Therefore, from a medical point of view, autophagy might as well be the key ingredient in solving some of the health concerns that have plagued society for years.

People who have diabetes, especially type-2 diabetes can also look up to autophagy since it has been proven effective in managing, if not reversing the effects and treating diabetes when detected early enough. This also works for those who are struggling with their blood sugar levels.

One area that has been highly controversial in recent times is dieting. There are a lot of fad diets that have been popular over the years, but barely help followers to meet their desired goals. Over time most of the people who start some of these diets end up slipping back into their former selves, and it can be so heartbreaking.

The problem that most of these diets have is that they have people doing many things without a proper perspective or initiative. Autophagy comes down to simple and easy to understand techniques for dieting. Diets like the ketogenic diet and intermittent fasting are key to realizing your autophagy goals.

If you take a closer look at these diets, you will realize that there is nothing very special about them. These are diets that can be followed by anyone, no matter their budgetary allocation or the condition they are living. These are diets that have you managing your life better with the food resources you have at your disposal.

A common concern that most people have with some diets is that you have to spend more to buy specific food items, some of which are exotic and might be very expensive for the average person. This is not the case with autophagy. This is one major factor that sets apart diet-induced autophagy and the fad diets that have been doing rounds all over the internet.

While still addressing the issue of dieting, another concern that people have is the inability to maintain their weight once they attain their desired weight. What is the purpose of struggling so hard to lose weight when you cannot keep it? This is a challenge that so many people struggle through. This also initiates a motion sequence that will, in the long run, open the door to anxiety and depression. The reason behind this is that no one ever prepares you for what comes after you have reached your target weight. For most people, everything ends when you get to your desired weight.

There are ways you can manage your life better, to maintain your weight. Of course, you have to be prepared for the fact that you might face challenges down the line, and you might put on some weight. However, simple procedures can help you manage your weight well, and avoid putting on more weight. Through autophagy, therefore, you are making effective changes in your life, loving the new changes, and keeping them.

Ultimately, everyone can optimize their body to induce autophagy. It is as simple as starting and following a diet that promotes autophagy. Whether you choose the intermittent fasting diet, ketogenic diet, water fasting or whichever diet that aligns with your goals, inducing autophagy might be the best decision you ever make.

Made in the USA
Lexington, KY
15 February 2019